PALEO BAKING

Paleo Cake Recipes

Table of Contents

Introduction

The biggest challenge for anyone when they hear the word diet, is resisting tasty and decadent sweets. Whether someone's favorite indulgence is fudgy chocolate cake, creamy coconut cream pie, ice cream, chocolate chip cookies or glazed donuts, sweets can be hard to resist when a craving strikes. So, is every healthy eating diet doomed to fail? Humans are wired to desire sweet foods because that is the easiest way to power our bodies. There is one diet plan that actually includes all these sweet treats, it's known as the Paleo diet. The Paleolithic diet takes the follower back to the age of the hunter/gatherers. It goes back to the caveman and cavewoman days, where the foods eaten were fruits, vegetables, meat, sea food and nuts. Well, nature happened to provide a delicious variety of naturally sweet foods that can be made into a healthy version of modern day favorites. Many nuts can be ground into flour-like substitutes that are just as delicious and without the negative impact to the body!

The possibilities of delicious and healthy cake recipes have arrived! Discover the variety of cakes that you can experiment with and find your favorite. Replace unhealthy, blood sugar spiking birthday, anniversary, holiday and even wedding cakes with the Paleo healthy alternative. It is surprising how delicious a healthy dessert can actually be. Plus, there is no guilt afterwards. When this diet is followed, research has shown a reduction in cholesterol, cardiovascular problems, blood pressure and body weight. The dieter will naturally replace empty calories with vitamins and minerals the body needs. Tie on that apron and crank up the oven, because here are delicious recipes to keep you busy for a while. You may convert your friends and family into modern day cavemen and woman with these scrumptious cakes!

Paleo Coconut Cake

Prep Time: 10 minutes

Cook Time: 25 minutes

Servings: 12

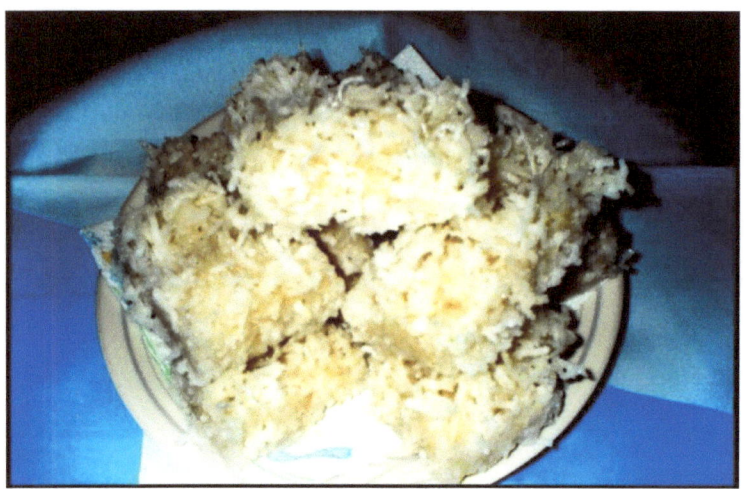

INGREDIENTS

Coconut Cake

6 cage-free eggs

3/4 cup coconut flour

1 cup flaked coconut

1 cup unsweetened applesauce

1/2 cup coconut oil

1/2 cup coconut milk

1/2 cup sweetener*

1/2 cup dried pitted dates

2 teaspoons vanilla

1 teaspoon baking soda

1 teaspoon baking powder

1/2 teaspoon Celtic sea salt

Coconut Frosting

1/3 cup coconut cream (from 1 can settled full-fat coconut milk)

2 - 4 tablespoons sweetener*

1/2 teaspoon vanilla

1/2 cup flaked coconut

INSTRUCTIONS

1. Preheat oven to 325°F. Line two or square baking pans with parchment or coat lightly with coconut oil.

2. Add dates, coconut milk, and half of eggs and oil to food processor or bullet blender. Process until dates a broken down, about 1 - 2 minutes.

3. Pour date mixture into medium bowl. Add applesauce, sweetener, vanilla, and remaining eggs and oil. Beat with hand mixer or whisk until well combined.

4. Sift coconut flour, salt, and baking soda and baking powder into wet ingredients. Blend until smooth. Stir in coconut.

5. Pour batter into prepared baking pans and bake for about 25 minutes, or until golden and toothpick inserted into center comes out clean.

6. Remove from oven and allow to cool. Place in refrigerator to speed cooling.

7. For *Coconut Frosting*, beat coconut cream in medium mixing bowl until slightly thickened. Add sweetener and vanilla, and continue to beat until full thickened and fluffy.

8. Frost cooled cakes and stack one on top of the other. Evenly sprinkle flaked coconut on top layer of frosted cake.
9. Slice and serve.

stevia, raw honey, agave nectar or maple syrup

Chocolate Zucchini Cake

Prep Time: 10 minutes

Cook Time: 25 minutes

Servings: 12

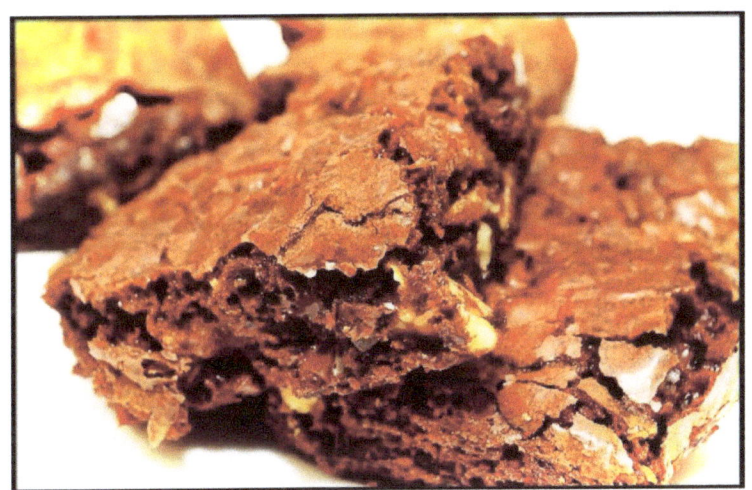

INGREDIENTS

1 1/2 cups almond flour

2 cage-free eggs

1 medium zucchini (1 1/2 cups grated)

1/2 cup unsweetened applesauce

1/4 cup coconut oil

1/4 - 1/2 cup sweetener*

1/4 cup cocoa powder

2 tablespoons ground chia seed (or flax meal)

1 teaspoon baking soda

1 teaspoon baking powder

1 teaspoon vanilla

1 teaspoon ground cinnamon

1 teaspoon ground black pepper

1/2 teaspoon Celtic sea salt

1/4 cup cocoa nibs or chocolate chips (optional)

INSTRUCTIONS

1. Preheat oven to 350 degrees F. Line rectangular baking pan with parchment or lightly coat with coconut oil.
2. Add eggs, coconut oil, applesauce and sweetener to food processor or bullet blender. Process until mixture is thick and lightened.
3. Grate zucchini and add to medium mixing bowl. Pour egg mixture over grated zucchini.
4. Sift almond flour, cocoa powder, chia meal, baking soda and powder, salt and spices into bowl. Beat with hand mixer or whisk to combine. Stir in cocoa nibs or chocolate chips (optional).
5. Pour batter into prepared baking pan and bake for about 25 minutes, until toothpick inserted into center comes out clean.
6. Remove from oven and let cool about 10 minutes.
7. Slice and serve warm. Or let cool completely and serve room temperature.

*stevia, raw honey or agave nectar

Paleo Pumpkin Bacon Cake

Prep Time: 15 minutes

Cook Time: 20 minutes

Servings: 12

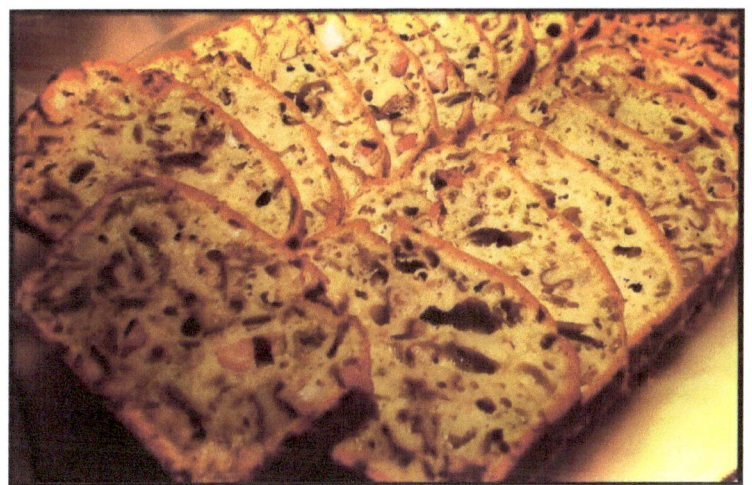

INGREDIENTS

3/4 cup coconut flour

4 cage-free eggs, separated

1/2 cup sweetener*

1/2 cup pumpkin purée

8 slices nitrate-free bacon

2 tablespoons coconut oil

1 teaspoon baking soda

1 teaspoon ground cinnamon

1/2 teaspoon ground black pepper

1/2 teaspoon vanilla

1/2 teaspoon Celtic sea salt

INSTRUCTIONS

1. Preheat oven to 350 degrees F. Line muffin pan with paper liners or lightly coat with coconut oil. Heat skillet over medium-high heat.
2. Finely chop bacon and add to hot skillet. Crisp bacon until fully cooked, about five minutes. Remove from heat.
3. Sift coconut flour, baking soda, salt and spices into large mixing bowl.
4. In medium mixing bowl, beat egg whites to soft peaks with a hand mixer or whisk. About 5 minutes.
5. Beat egg yolks, oil, sweetener and pumpkin purée into egg whites. Add yolk mixture to dry ingredient and mix well. Pour in bacon and drippings and mix until combined.
6. Pour batter into prepared muffin pan and bake 20 - 25 minutes, or until firm but springy in the center. Toothpick insert into the middle should come out clean.
7. Remove from oven and let cool about 10 minutes.
8. Serve warm. Or cool completely and serve room temperature.

NOTE: For large **Pumpkin Bacon Cake**, oil large loaf pan or square baking pan and bake 45 minutes.

* raw honey, agave nectar or maple syrup

Caveman German Chocolate Cake

Prep Time: 10 minutes

Cook Time: 15 minutes

Servings: 12

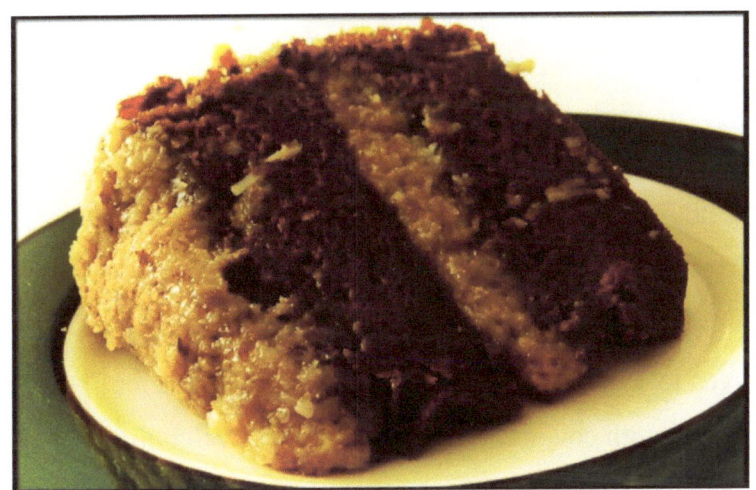

INGREDIENTS

Chocolate Cake

6 cage-free eggs

1 cup coconut flour

1/2 cup cocoa powder

1/2 cup coconut oil

1/2 cup sweetener

1/2 cup applesauce

1/2 cup dried pitted dates

1 cup water

2 teaspoons vanilla

1 teaspoon baking soda

1 teaspoon Celtic sea salt

1/4 teaspoon ground black pepper (optional)

Coconut Pecan Topping

3/4 cup flaked or shredded coconut

1/2 cup pecans

1/2 cup full-fat coconut milk

1/2 cup sweetener*

1/2 teaspoon vanilla

Pinch Celtic sea salt

INSTRUCTIONS

1. Preheat oven to 350 degrees F. Line muffin pan with paper liners or lightly coat with coconut oil. Bring 1 cup water to boil in small pan.
2. Add dried dates to boiling water for about 5 minutes.
3. For *Chocolate Cake*, sift flour, cocoa, baking soda, salt and pepper (optional) into small bowl.
4. In medium bowl, beat eggs until thick and frothy, about 5 minutes.
5. Add dates with just enough hot water to food processor or bullet blender to process into thick paste.
6. Add date paste, sweetener, applesauce, coconut oil and vanilla to eggs. Beat with hand mixer or whisk until combined.
7. Beat flour mixture into egg mixture until well combined.
8. Use ice cream scoop or spoon to pour batter into prepared muffin pan.
9. Place in oven and bake about 15 minutes, or until center is set but springy. Toothpick inserted into center should come out clean.

10. Heat small pan over medium heat.

11. For *Coconut Pecan Topping*, chop pecans and add to hot dry pan. Stir and toast pecans about 5 minutes, careful not to burn.

12. Add toasted pecans to small bowl with coconut, sweetener, coconut milk, vanilla and salt. Mix until well combined. Mixture should be thick and gooey.

13. Remove muffin pan from oven and let cool about 10 minutes.

14. Frost cakes with *Coconut Pecan Topping*.

15. Serve warm. Or allow to cool completely and serve room temperature.

NOTE: For large **German Chocolate Cake**, bake in square baking pan for 40 - 45 minutes.

* raw honey, agave nectar or maple syrup

Primal Lemon Coconut Cake

Prep Time: 10 minutes

Cook Time: 30 minutes

Servings: 12

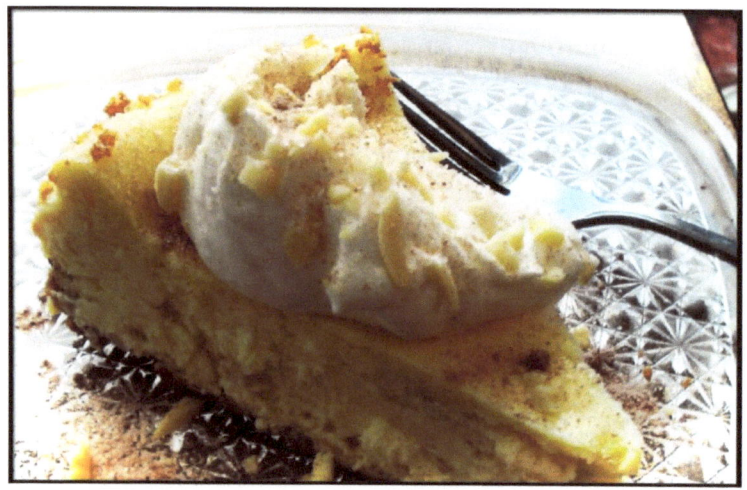

INGREDIENTS

Lemon Coconut Cake

6 cage-free eggs

3/4 cup coconut flour

1 cup flaked or shredded coconut

1/2 cup unsweetened applesauce

1/2 cup lemon juice (about 5 lemons)

1/2 cup sweetener*

1/2 cup dried pitted dates

1/2 cup coconut milk

1/4 cup coconut oil

1 teaspoon vanilla

1 teaspoon baking soda

1 teaspoon baking powder

1/2 teaspoon Celtic sea salt

Lemon Coconut Icing

1/2 cup flaked or shredded coconut

1/3 cup full-fat coconut milk

1/3 cup sweetener**

Juice of 1 lemon

1/4 teaspoon vanilla

INSTRUCTIONS

10. Preheat oven to 325 degrees F. Line square baking pan with parchment or lightly coat with coconut oil.

11. Add dates, coconut milk, oil and 3 eggs to food processor or bullet blender. Process until dates break down, about 1 - 2 minutes.

12. Pour date mixture into medium bowl. Add applesauce, sweetener, lemon juice, vanilla, and remaining eggs. Beat with hand mixer or whisk until well combined.

13. Sift coconut flour, salt, baking soda and baking powder into wet ingredients. Blend until smooth. Stir in coconut.

14. Pour batter into prepared baking pan and bake for about 30 minutes, or until golden brown and toothpick inserted into center comes out clean.

15. Remove from oven and allow to cool. Place in refrigerator to speed cooling.

16. For *Lemon Coconut Icing*, beat coconut milk, sweetener, lemon juice and vanilla in small bowl until well combined. Mixture should be fairly thin and runny.

17. Coat *Lemon Coconut Cake* with *Lemon Coconut Icing*. Sprinkle on coconut.

18. Slice and serve warm. Or allow to cool completely and serve room temperature.

*stevia, raw honey or agave nectar

**raw honey, agave nectar or maple syrup

Flourless Chocolate Cake

Prep Time: 15 minutes

Cook Time: 30 minutes

Servings: 8

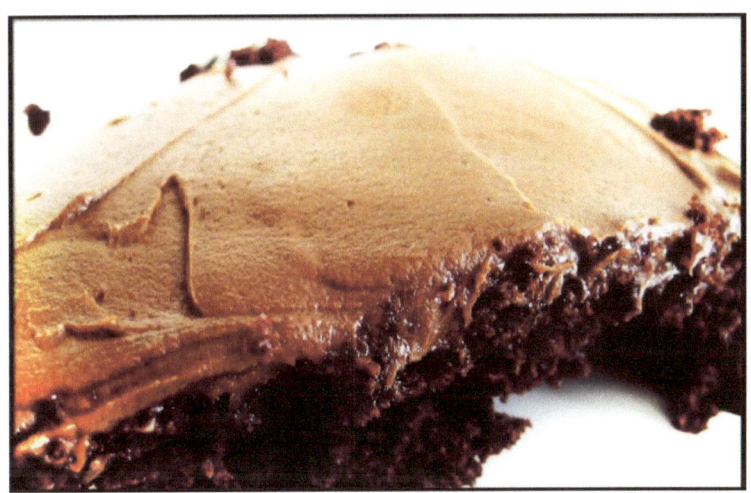

INGREDIENTS

16 oz organic bittersweet chocolate

1/4 cup cocoa powder

6 cage-free eggs

1 cup coconut oil

3/4 cup sweetener*

2 tablespoons water

2 teaspoons vanilla

1/4 teaspoon Celtic sea salt

INSTRUCTIONS

1. Preheat oven to 275 degrees F. Coat 2 mini springform pans with coconut oil, then dust with cocoa powder, and cover the outside base of the pans with aluminum foil. Or line muffin pan with paper liners, or leave bare and coat liners or bare pan with coconut oil and dust with cocoa powder.

2. Slowly melt chocolate and coconut oil over a double boiler, heated over medium heat. Do not boil water in bottom of double boiler. Stir frequently.

3. Remove from heat once chocolate is melted and beat in sweetener, water, vanilla, salt and any remaining cocoa powder with hand mixer or whisk.

4. Beat in eggs one at a time until thoroughly incorporated.

5. Pour batter into vessels and bake for about 25 - 30 minutes, until set. Cakes will still appear a bit glossy and wet in the middle.

6. Cool for 30 minutes, then refrigerate at least 2 hours before serving.

7. Cut springform cakes with a knife warmed until hot running water, then dried.

8. Serve chilled or room temperature.

*maple syrup, raw honey or agave nectar

Pumpkin Spice Cakes

Prep Time: 5 minutes

Cook Time: 15 minutes

Servings: 12

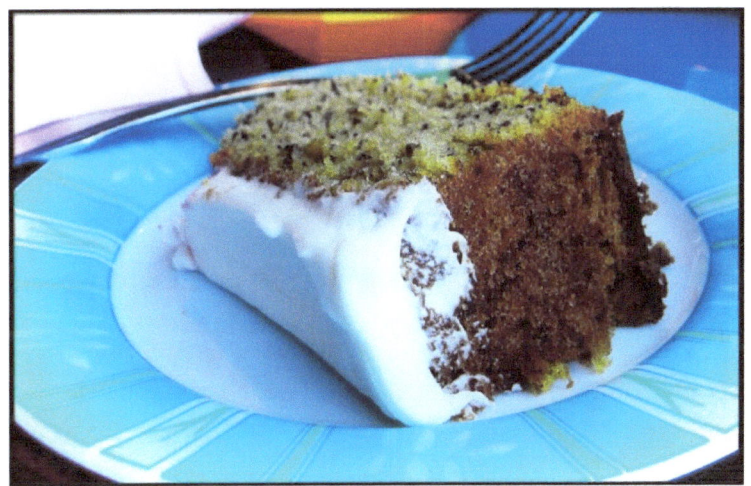

INGREDIENTS

3/4 cup coconut flour

4 cage-free eggs

1/4 cup coconut oil

1/2 cup sweetener*

1/2 cup pumpkin purée

1 teaspoon baking soda

1 tablespoon ground cinnamon

1 tablespoon ground ginger

1 tablespoon ground nutmeg

1 tablespoon ground black pepper

1 teaspoon vanilla

1/2 teaspoon Celtic sea salt

1/4 cup pumpkin seeds

INSTRUCTIONS

1. Preheat oven to 350 degrees F. Lightly coat 4 mini cake pans or mini loaf pans with coconut oil, or line with parchment paper.
2. Sift coconut flour, baking soda, salt and spices into large mixing bowl.
3. In medium mixing bowl, beat egg whites to soft peaks with hand mixer or whisk. About 5 minutes.
4. Then beat in yolks, oil, sweetener and pumpkin purée. Mix wet ingredients into dry blend until combined.
5. Pour batter into mini cake loaf pans and sprinkle on pumpkin seeds.
6. Bake for 20 - 25 minutes, or until firm but springy in the center and browned. A toothpick inserted into the middle should come out clean.
7. Remove from oven and allow to cool for 5 minutes before serving.
8. Serve warm or room temperature.

NOTE: For large **Pumpkin Spice Cake**, oil large loaf pan or springform pan and bake 40 - 45 minutes.

raw honey, agave nectar or maple syrup

Fruit and Nut Cake

Prep Time: 10 minutes

Cook Time: 25 minutes

Servings: 8

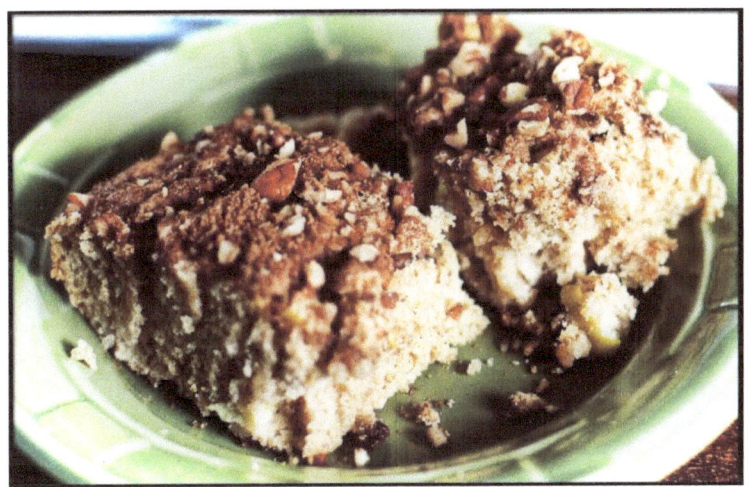

INGREDIENTS

1 1/2 cup almond flour

4 cage-free eggs

2 tablespoons coconut oil

Juice of orange half

1/4 cup sweetener*

1/2 cup walnuts

1/4 cup pecans

1/2 cup dried pitted dates

1/2 cup dried cherries

1/4 cup dried apricots

1/4 cup raisins

1/2 teaspoon baking soda

1 teaspoon ground ginger

1 teaspoon vanilla

1/2 teaspoon Celtic sea salt

Zest of orange half

INSTRUCTIONS

1. Preheat oven to 350 degrees F. Lightly coat 2 small loaf pans or one Bundt pan with coconut oil.
2. Sift almond flour, baking soda and salt into large mixing bowl.
3. Chop walnuts, pecans, apricots and dates. Then stir all dried fruit and nuts into flour mixture.
4. In medium mixing bowl, mix eggs, coconut oil, juice and zest of half an orange, sweetener, ginger and vanilla. Then pour and mix into dry ingredients until just combined.
5. Scoop batter into loaf pans or Bundt pan, and smooth tops with spatula.
6. Bake 20 - 30 minutes, or until firm, browned and firm in the center.
7. Remove from oven and allow to cool before slicing.
8. Serve warm or room temperature.

*stevia, raw honey or agave nectar

Toasted Almond Cream Cakes

Prep Time: 15 minutes*

Cook Time: 20 minutes

Servings: 12

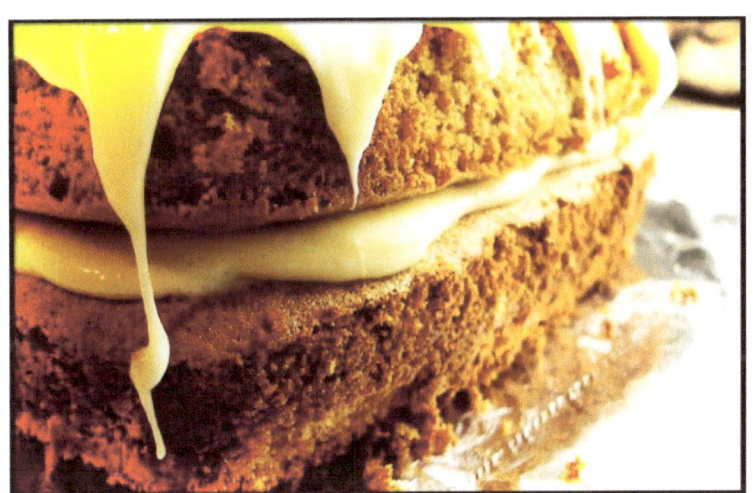

INGREDIENTS

Cake

1 cup almond flour

4 cage-free egg whites

1/3 cup coconut oil

1/4 cup almond milk

1/4 cup sweetener*

1 teaspoon baking powder

1/4 cup slice almonds

Almond Cream

2 cups skinless almonds

1/4 cup sweetener

1 teaspoon vanilla

Water

INSTRUCTIONS

1. *Soak almonds overnight in water. Drain and rinse.
2. Preheat the oven to 350 degrees F. Heat medium pan over medium heat. Lightly coat muffin pan with coconut oil, or line with paper liners
3. Add almond flour to hot dry pan and toast about 5 minutes, stirring frequently. Do not burn. Remove from heat and set aside.
4. Beat egg whites to soft peaks with hand mixer or whisk in medium bowl. Then beat in oil, milk and 1/4 cup sweetener. Sift in toasted almond flour and baking powder. Mix until just combined.
5. Use ice cream scoop or spoon to scoop batter into muffin pan. Each cup should be only 1/2 full.
6. Bake about 15 minutes, or until center is set but springy.
7. Remove pan from oven and remove cakes from pan. Let cool for about 15 minutes.
8. While cakes cool, blend soaked almonds, 1/4 cup sweetener, 1 teaspoon vanilla and water as needed in food processor or blender to make smooth *Almond Cream.*
9. Wipe out pan with paper towel and return dry pan to medium heat. Toast slice almonds about 5 minutes, until aromatic and golden. Do not burn. Remove from heat and set aside.
10. When cakes are cooled, slice in half to create top and bottom layer. Scoop cream onto bottom half, and top with top half of cake.

Scoop another dollop of cream over top half and sprinkle on slice toasted almonds.

11. Serve room temperature.

NOTE: For large **Toasted Almond Cream Cake** , bake batter in 2 round cake pans for 35 - 40 minutes.

* raw honey, agave nectar or maple syrup

Pineapple Upside Down Cake

Prep Time: 15 minutes

Cook Time: 30 minutes

Servings: 12

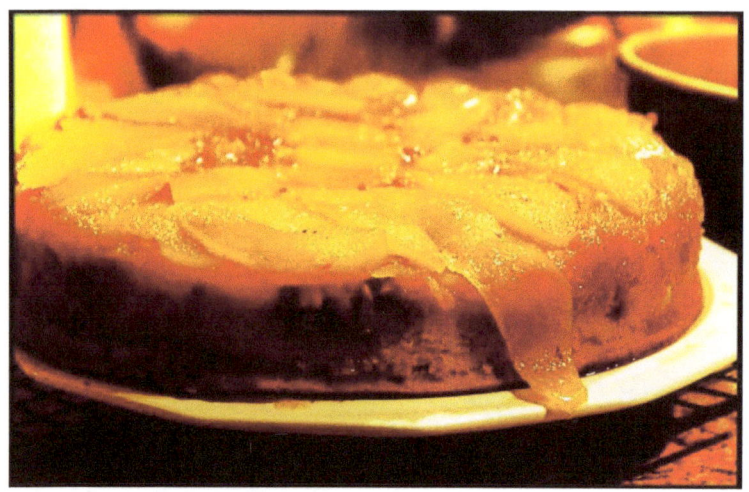

INGREDIENTS

2 cups almond flour

8 - 12 slices organic canned pineapple in juice

8 - 12 pitted cherries

1/4 cup sweetener*

3 cage-free eggs

1/4 cup coconut oil

1/2 cup organic pineapple juice (reserved from can)

2 teaspoons baking soda

2 teaspoons vanilla

1/2 teaspoon Celtic sea salt

INSTRUCTIONS

1. Preheat oven to 350 degrees F. Line 9x13 baking dish with parchment paper, or coat with coconut oil.

2. Arrange pineapple slices and cherries on bottom of baking dish. Place in oven while you prepare the batter.

3. Beat egg whites to stiff peaks with hand mixer or whisk in medium mixing bowl. About 7 - 10 minutes.

4. In large mixing bowl, mix yolks, olive oil, sweetener, pineapple juice and vanilla.

5. Sift almond flour, baking soda and salt into yolk mixture. Beat until well combined.

6. Fold egg whites into batter until evenly combined.

7. Remove hot baking pan from oven, and spread light batter over pineapple and cherries. Smooth top with spatula.

8. Bake for 25 - 30 minutes, or until cake golden brown and firm but springy in the center. A toothpick inserted into the center should come out clean.

9. Remove pan from oven and allow to cool for 15 minutes. Turn cake out onto serving dish and remove parchment. Or scrape any stuck fruit from the pan and place back on cake.

10. Allow to cool another 15 minutes before serving. Serve room temperature or warm.

NOTE: For **Pineapple Upside Dow Cupcakes** , add a pineapple slice and cherry to muffin pan lined with paper liners or coated with coconut oil, then fill cups 2/3 full with batter and bake about 20 minutes.

*stevia, raw honey or agave nectar

Paleo Cocoa-nut Cake

Prep Time: 10 minutes

Cook Time: 25 minutes

Servings: 12

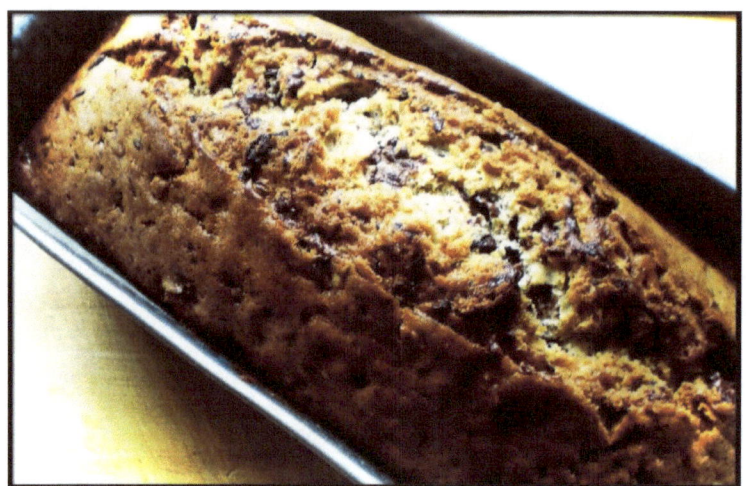

INGREDIENTS

Chocolate Coconut Cake

3/4 cup coconut flour

6 cage-free eggs

1 cup flaked or shredded coconut

1 cup unsweetened applesauce

1/2 cup coconut oil

1/2 cup coconut milk

1/2 cup sweetener*

1/2 cup dried pitted dates

1/3 cup cocoa powder

1 teaspoon vanilla

1 teaspoon baking soda

1 teaspoon baking powder

1/2 teaspoon Celtic sea salt

Chocolate Coconut Topping

Coconut cream (settled from 1 can full-fat coconut milk)

2 - 4 tablespoons sweetener*

2 tablespoons cocoa powder

1/2 teaspoon vanilla

1/2 cup flaked or shredded coconut

INSTRUCTIONS

1. Preheat oven to 325 degrees F. Line two round or square baking pans with parchment or lightly coat with coconut oil.

2. For *Chocolate Coconut Cake*, add dates, coconut milk, and half of eggs and oil to food processor or high-speed blender. Process until fairly smooth, about 1 - 2 minutes.

3. Pour date mixture into medium bowl. Add applesauce, sweetener, vanilla, and remaining eggs and oil. Beat with hand mixer or whisk until well combined.

4. Sift coconut flour, cocoa, salt, and baking soda and powder into wet ingredients. Blend until smooth. Stir in coconut.

5. Divide batter and pour into prepared baking pans and bake for about 25 minutes, or until golden and toothpick inserted into center comes out clean.

6. For *Chocolate Coconut Topping*, beat coconut cream in medium mixing bowl until slightly thickened. Add sweetener, vanilla and cocoa. Continue to beat until fully thickened and fluffy.

7. Remove cakes from oven and allow to cool. Place in refrigerator to speed cooling.

8. Frost cooled cakes and stack one on top of the other. Evenly sprinkle flaked coconut over top layer.

9. Slice and serve.

stevia, raw honey, agave nectar or maple syrup

Paleo Chocolate Truffles

Prep Time: 20 minutes*

Cook Time: 5 minutes

Servings: 12

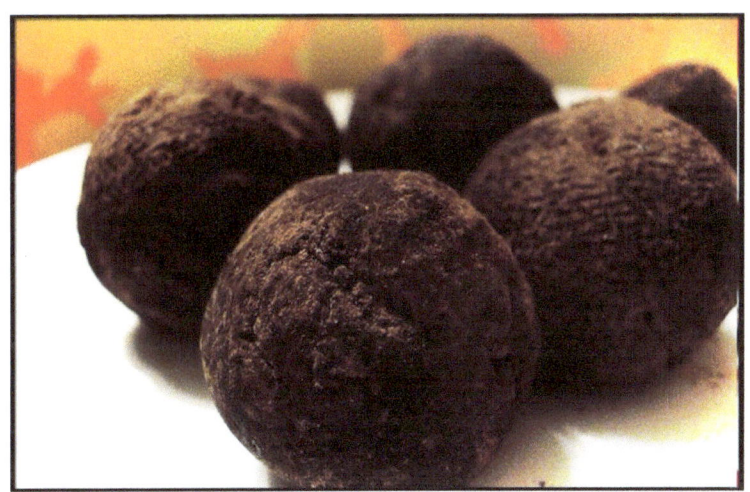

INGREDIENTS

1/4 cup cocoa powder

1 cup almond butter (or 1 1/2 cup almonds)

2 tablespoons coconut oil

1/4 cup sweetener**

1/2 teaspoon vanilla

2 - 4 tablespoons cocoa powder

INSTRUCTIONS

1. Line square baking dish with parchment paper.

2. To make nut butter, process almonds and coconut oil in food processor or bullet blender until smooth. Let mixture rest, then continue processing if necessary.

3. Add almond butter to small bowl with 1/4 cup cocoa powder, sweetener and vanilla. Mix well.

4. *Spread mixture into parchment lined baking dish and place in freezer for about 20 minutes if mixture is too soft to form balls.

5. Use melon baller or mini scoop to make 12 balls from mixture. Roll in hands to make uniform if necessary.

6. Add cocoa powder to shallow dish and roll truffles in cocoa powder to coat.

7. Place *Paleo Chocolate Truffles* in refrigerator for 20 minutes.

8. Serve chilled.

** raw honey, agave nectar or maple syrup

Caveman Chocolate Macaroons

Prep Time: 10 minutes

Cook Time: 20 minutes

Servings: 18

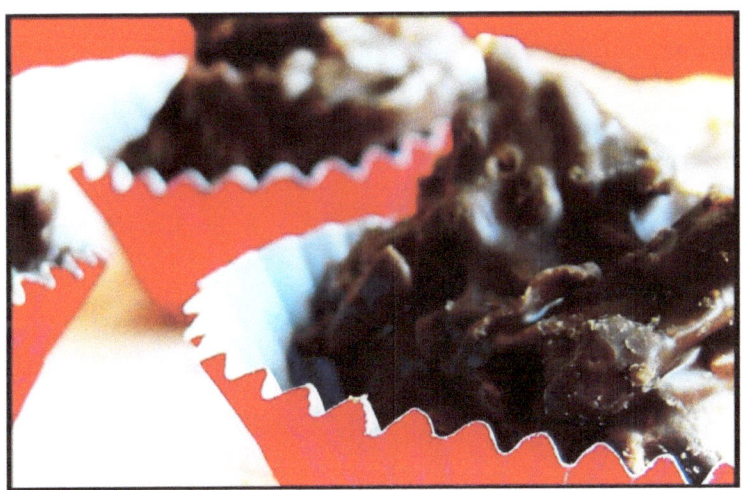

INGREDIENTS

6 cage-free egg whites

3 cups flaked or shredded coconut

1/2 cup sweetener*

1/4 cup cocoa powder

1 tablespoon coconut oil

1 tablespoon vanilla

1/4 teaspoon Celtic sea salt

1/4 teaspoon cinnamon (optional)

INSTRUCTIONS

1. Preheat oven to 350 degrees F. Line sheet pan with parchment paper or baking mat.
2. In medium mixing bowl, beat room temperature egg whites and salt to stiff peaks with hand mixer or stand mixer, about 7 - 8 minutes.
3. Beat in sweetener, cocoa, vanilla and cinnamon (optional) until combined. Fold in coconut 1 cup at a time.
4. Use scoop or tablespoon to drop portions of batter onto prepared sheet pan.
5. Bake for 15 - 17 minutes, or until coconut is toasted and cookies are set.
6. Allow to cool for 10 minutes, then transfer to wire rack to cool completely.
7. Serve room temperature.

*stevia, raw honey or agave nectar

Paleo Coconut Macaroons

Prep Time: 10 minutes

Cook Time: 20 minutes

Servings: 12

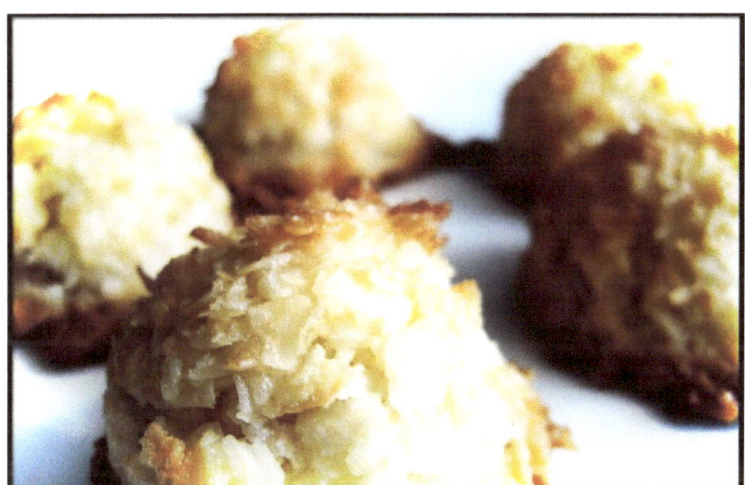

INGREDIENTS

6 cage-free egg whites

3 cups flaked coconut

1/2 cup sweetener*

1 tablespoon coconut oil

1 teaspoon vanilla

1/4 teaspoon Celtic sea salt

INSTRUCTIONS

1. Preheat oven to 350 degrees F. Line a sheet pan with parchment
   paper or baking mat.

2. In large mixing bowl, beat room temperature egg whites with hand mixer to stiff peaks, about 7 - 8 minutes.

3. Beat in sweetener, vanilla and salt until combined. Fold in 1 cup of coconut at a time.

4. Use ice cream scoop or spoon to drop rounds of batter onto prepared sheet pan.

5. Bake for about 20 minutes, or until coconut is toasted and browned.

6. Allow to cool on pan for 10 minutes. Then remove from pan.

7. Serve warm. Or allow to cool completely and serve room temperature.

raw honey or agave nectar

Lemon Poppy Seed Muffins

Prep Time: 5 minutes

Cook Time: 20 minutes

Servings: 12

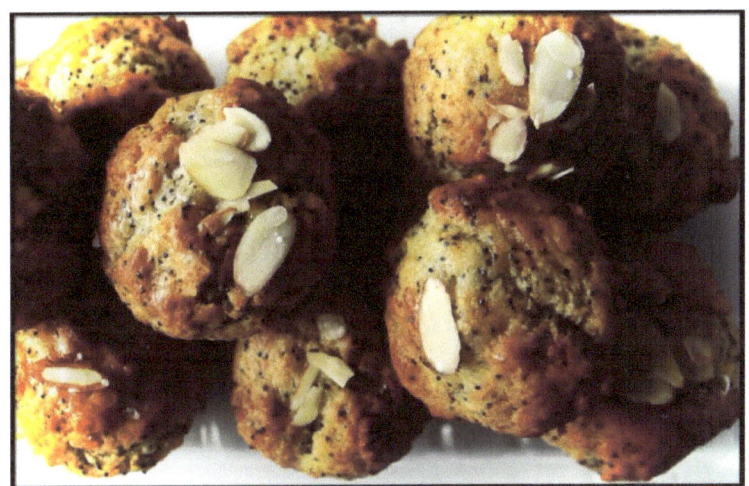

INGREDIENTS

6 cage-free eggs

1/2 cup coconut flour

1/4 cup coconut oil

1/4 cup sweetener*

1 teaspoon vanilla

1 teaspoon poppy seeds

1/2 teaspoon baking soda

Juice of 2 lemons

Zest of 2 lemons

INSTRUCTIONS

1. Preheat oven to 350 degrees F. Oil muffin pan or line with paper liners.
2. Zest, *then* juice 2 lemons. Add to large mixing bowl with eggs, coconut oil, sweetener and vanilla. Beat with hand mixer or whisk until well combined.
3. Sift coconut flour and baking soda into wet ingredients, and mix until smooth. Stir in poppy seeds.
4. Use ice cream scoop or tablespoon to pour batter into prepared muffin pan.
5. Place in oven and bake for about 20 minutes, or until golden around edges and toothpick inserted into middle comes out clean.
6. Remove from oven and let cool for 5 minutes.
7. Serve warm. Or allow to cool completely and serve room temperature.

* raw honey or agave nectar

Cocoa Cream Muffins

Prep Time: 10 minutes*

Cook Time: 20 minutes

Servings: 12

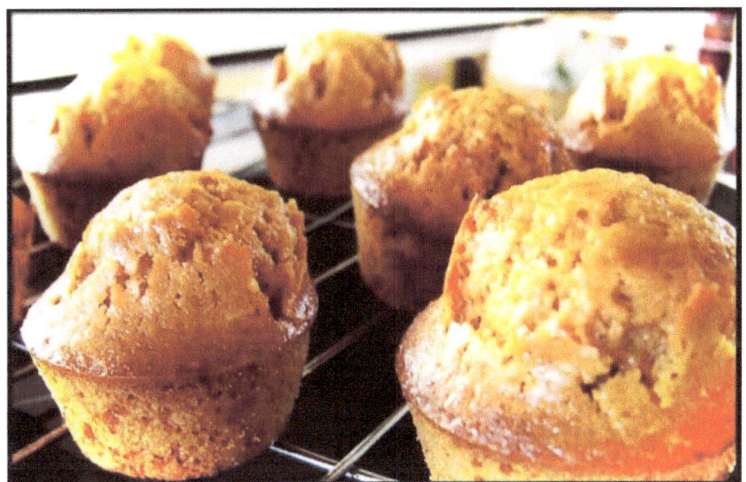

INGREDIENTS

1 cup almond flour

1 cup coconut flour

3 cage-free eggs

1/2 cup unsweetened applesauce

1/4 cup coconut oil

1/4 cup sweetener*

1 avocado

3 tablespoons cocoa powder

1 tablespoon baking powder

1/4 teaspoon ground black pepper

1 teaspoon Celtic sea salt

Filling

2 cups water

1 cup cashews

3 tablespoons sweetener*

2 tablespoon cocoa powder

2 - 4 tablespoons coconut milk

INSTRUCTIONS

1. *Soak cashews overnight in 2 cups water. Drain and rinse. Set aside.
2. Preheat oven to 350 degrees F. Line muffin pan with paper liners or coat with coconut oil.
3. Slice avocado in half, pit, and scoop flesh into food processor or blender. Add eggs, coconut oil, applesauce and sweetener. Process until smooth.
4. Pour avocado blend into medium mixing bowl. Sift in almond flour, cocoa powder, baking powder, salt and pepper. Beat with hand mixer or whisk until combined.
5. Pour batter into prepared muffin pan. Bake 20 -25 minutes, or until firm but springy in center.
6. For *Filling*, add soaked cashews, sweetener and cocoa powder to food processor or bullet blender. Process until smooth and creamy. Add coconut milk if necessary to reach desired consistency.
7. Remove muffins from oven and let cool.
8. Scoop out center of muffin with knife or teaspoon, and fill with *Filling*. Or transfer *Filling* to pastry bag fitted with 1/2 inch tip, insert tip into muffin and fill.

9. Serve warm or room temperature.

*stevia, raw honey or agave nectar

Orange Cranberry Muffins

Prep Time: 5 minutes

Cook Time: 20 minutes

Servings: 12

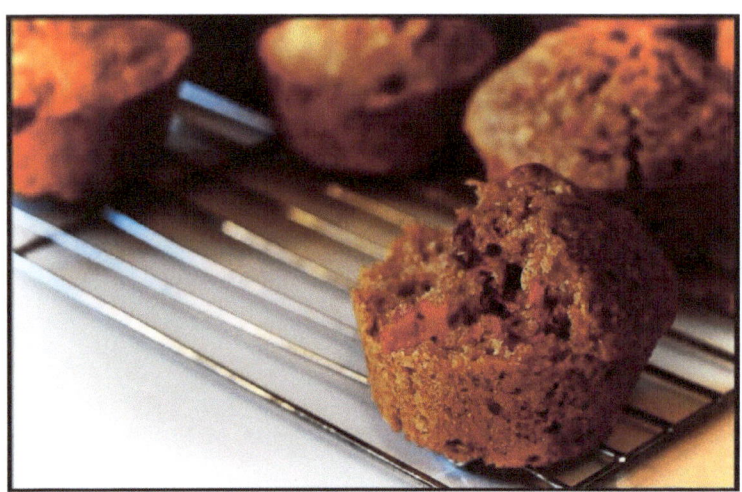

INGREDIENTS

1 1/2 cups almond flour

2 cage-free eggs

1/2 cup fresh squeezed orange juice (about 2 oranges)

1/4 cup coconut oil

1/4 cup dried cranberries

1 tablespoon orange zest

1 teaspoon baking powder

1/2 teaspoon vanilla

1/2 teaspoon Celtic sea salt

INSTRUCTIONS

1. Preheat oven to 350 degrees F. Line muffin pan with paper liners or coconut oil.

2. In medium bowl, beat eggs with hand mixer or whisk until light and a foamy. Add coconut oil, orange juice and zest. Beat well.

3. Sift in almond flour, baking powder, vanilla and salt. Mix until combined. Stir in cranberries.

4. Use ice cream scoop or tablespoon to scoop batter into prepared muffin pan.

5. Bake about 20 minutes, or until toothpick inserted into center comes out clean.

6. Remove from oven and serve warm. Or let cool completely and serve room temperature.

NOTE: Bake in oiled loaf pan for 40 - 45 minutes for **Cranberry Orange Bread**.

stevia, raw honey or agave nectar

Double Pumpkin Muffins

Prep Time: 5 minutes

Cook Time: 25 minutes

Servings: 12

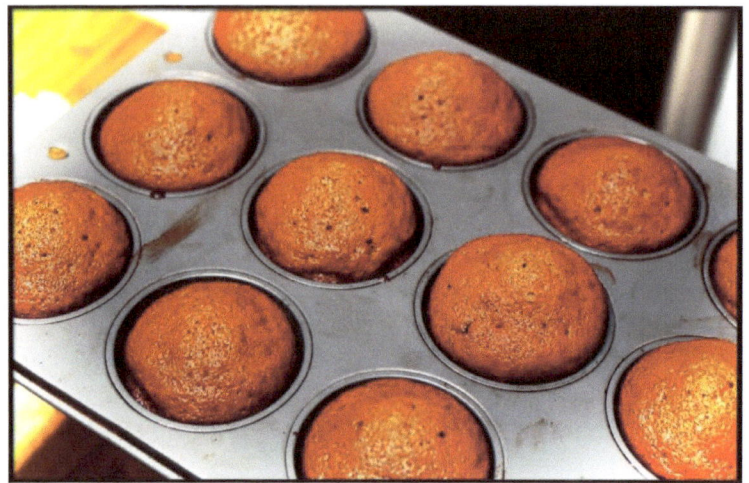

INGREDIENTS

1 3/4 cups coconut flour

2 cage-free eggs

15 oz (1 can) organic pumpkin puree

1 cup unsweetened applesauce

1/2 cup coconut oil

1/4 cup sweetener*

2 teaspoons baking soda

1 1/2 tablespoon ground cinnamon

1/2 teaspoon ground nutmeg

1 teaspoon Celtic sea salt

1/2 cup pumpkin seeds

INSTRUCTIONS

1. Preheat oven to 350 degrees F. Line muffin pan with paper liner or coat with coconut oil.

2. Process eggs, coconut oil, applesauce and sweetener in food processor or blender until thick and light, about 2 minutes.

3. Pour egg mixture into medium mixing bowl. Add pumpkin puree, salt and spices and mix with hand mixer or whisk.

4. Sift in coconut flour and baking soda. Mix until well combined. Stir in half of pumpkin seeds.

5. Pour batter into prepared muffin pan and sprinkle remaining pumpkin seeds over batter.

6. Place in oven and bake 20 - 25 minutes , until edges are golden and tops firm but springy.

7. Remove from oven and allow to cool 5 minutes.

8. Serve warm. Or let cool complete and serve room temperature.

*stevia, raw honey or agave nectar

Paleo Avocado Club Muffin

Prep Time: 10 minutes

Cook Time: 15 minutes

Servings: 12

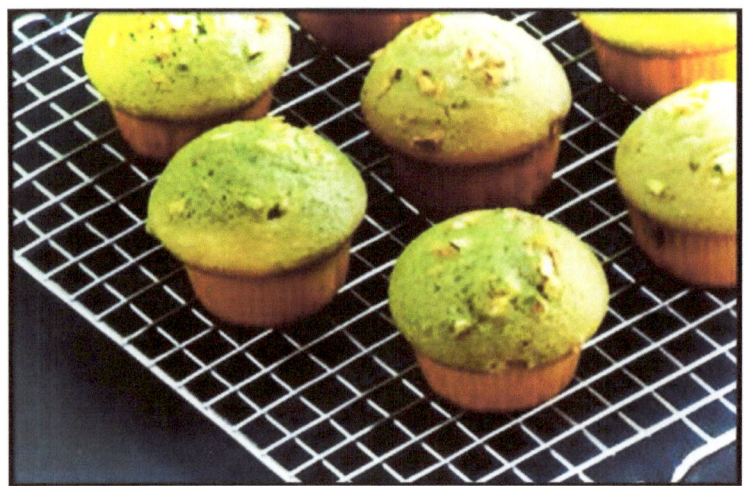

INGREDIENTS

1 cup almond flour

2 cage-free eggs

1 avocado

4 slices nitrate-free bacon

1 tablespoon sweetener*

1 teaspoon apple cider vinegar

1 teaspoon baking powder

1/4 teaspoon ground white pepper (or black pepper)

INSTRUCTIONS

1. Preheat oven to 350 degrees F. Line muffin pan with paper liners or light coat with coconut oil. Heat medium pan over medium-high heat.
2. Finely chop bacon and add to hot pan. Sauté until crisp and cooked through, about 5 minutes. Set aside.
3. Beat eggs, sweetener and vinegar in medium mixing bowl with hand mixer or whisk until thick and slightly foamy.
4. Slice avocado in half. Scoop flesh of one half into egg mixture. Add bacon and drippings, almond flour, baking powder and black pepper and mix until combined.
5. Dice remaining avocado flesh and fold into batter.
6. Use ice cream scoop or tablespoon to scoop batter into prepared muffin pan.
7. Bake about 15 - 20 minutes, until edges are golden brown and tops are firm.
8. Remove from oven and let cool for 5 minutes.
9. Serve warm. Or cool completely and serve temperature.

NOTE: Bake in square oiled baking pan for 30 - 35 minutes for **Avocado Club Bread**.

stevia, raw honey or agave nectar